1

Cancer: A Great Concern for Thyroid Patients

Malignancies Affecting the Metabolic Butterfly

By: James M. Lowrance © 2011

TABLE OF CONTENTS:

INTRODUCTION:

According to some medical information sources, thyroid disease is the most common of the endocrine diseases, including diabetes.

This is what the American Association of Clinical Endocrinologists (AACE) has to say about it:

"Thyroid disease is more common than diabetes or heart disease. Thyroid disease is a fact of life for as many as 27 million Americans – and more than half of those people remain undiagnosed." (From Their "Empower" Website)
Source Link:
http://www.empoweryourhealth.org/thyroid-conditions)

Many thyroid disease patients become aware of the fact that they are at an increased risk for developing thyroid malignancy but they are unsure how much that risk increases following diagnosis of their thyroid condition. Within the chapters of this book that follow, I offer information regarding these increased risk factors, backed by reputable medical information sources.

Also included is information regarding thyroid cancer prevention, detection and treatments.

I believe this information may offer some comfort to thyroid disease patients but it will also help them to know what to look for regarding signs and symptoms of these higher-risk diseases and possibly to know what blood tests or other medical evaluations they may wish to request from their doctors should they suspect the possible onset of a malignant thyroid disease. I am including quotes from medical research studies found on the U.S. National Institutes of Health website (reprints allowed for educational purposes).

Being aware of the medical possibilities and how they may manifest, through self-education, is part of what we in Thyroid Patient Advocacy refer-to as being "a proactive thyroid patient" and by doing so, one can help to secure a better quality of life for the sake of their selves and their families.

-*Jim Lowrance*

CHAPTER ONE

Can My Thyroid Disease Lead to Cancer in the Gland?

Most people who develop either hypothyroidism (underactive gland) or hyperthyroidism (overactive gland), do so as a result of "thyroid autoimmunity". This is the term that refers to the process in which auto-antibodies (destructive cells), attack the thyroid gland, rendering it incapable of producing proper amounts of thyroid hormone, to regulate metabolism within the cells of the body (the rate at which the body processes fuels coming into it for energy).

Some research studies have shown an increased risk by people who have Grave's disease, for developing thyroid cancer of which the most common types are "follicular" and "papillary" malignancies ("medullary" and "anaplastic" are the less common types).

Following is a research study excerpt, published by the U.S. National Institutes of Health (PubMed), in regard to this risk:

Cancer: A Great Concern for Thyroid Patients

"The relationship between Graves' disease or its therapy and carcinoma of the thyroid remains uncertain. We studied 20 patients found to have thyroid cancer in glands previously treated for Graves' disease between 1961 and 1986 at the University of Chicago Medical Center. Sixteen (80%) occurred in women and four (20%) occurred in men. The mean age at operation was 37 years (range, 19 to 69 years) and did not differ by sex. Fifteen of the 20 cancers (75%) were papillary while five (25%) were follicular. Six individuals (30%) had a history of external radiation to the head and neck as an infant, child, or young adult. Two others had received radioiodine (RAI) therapy for Graves' disease 1 and 19 years earlier.

Patients were divided into three groups: group I: four patients (20%) had a neck mass 4, 14, 20, and 41 years after having had a subtotal thyroidectomy (STT) for Graves' disease; three of four had a history of external irradiation therapy. These tumors behaved aggressively, resulting in the death of two of the four patients. group II: 11 patients (55%) had diffusely enlarge toxic goiters without a nodule. ---

Cancer: A Great Concern for Thyroid Patients

A carcinoma was diagnosed intraoperatively on frozen section in only two of these patients. The others received STT. After recognition on permanent section, those carcinomas that were 4 mm or greater in diameter received postoperative RAI.

One recurrence occurred and was treated successfully with further RAI. group III: Five patients (25%) had Graves' disease and a palpable thyroid nodule. None of them had had a prior thyroidectomy for Graves' disease, as in group 1. Thyroid carcinoma was diagnosed in all patients preoperatively or intraoperatively, and a total thyroidectomy was performed. Each patient is alive and well with a mean follow-up of 5 years.

Between 1971 and 1981, 194 patients had surgery for Graves' disease, and 10 (5.2%) were found to have an associated carcinoma; six patients (3.1% of the total) did not have a nodule or any other suspicion of malignancy before surgery. During the same time, 303 patients received RAI therapy for Graves' disease and one (0.3%) has subsequently developed thyroid carcinoma. ---

Cancer: A Great Concern for Thyroid Patients

Thyroid cancer associated with Graves' disease is found more commonly in surgically treated patients than in patients after RAI therapy.

The greatest risk factor in our patients was previous external radiation to the head and neck. Such individuals should be treated with total thyroid ablation rather than the usual STT, since they are at risk of developing aggressive thyroid cancers if thyroid remnants are left."

Source Link:
http://www.ncbi.nlm.nih.gov/pubmed/3787468
("Graves' disease and thyroid cancer.")

This particular study states that the risk for cancer in Graves' patients was more highly increased in those who underwent surgical subtotal thyroidectomies (SST -- partial removal of their glands), as opposed to those who had their thyroid glands ablated (destruction of it through radioactive iodine administration). The research also points-out that the history of a significant percent of patient-participants in the study who developed thyroid cancer associated with their Graves' disease, had a history of external head and neck radiation as infants.

Cancer: A Great Concern for Thyroid Patients

This was during their childhoods, or during young adulthood (possibly referring mainly to frequent x-rays).

Other Studies have shown an increased risk for ovarian cancer in women with Graves' disease as well.

A similar study published on the U.S. NIH, PubMed website, states that people with Hashimoto's disease (autoimmune thyroiditis that leads to hypothyroidism), are also at increased risk for developing thyroid cancer of the "papillary type" and that this risk is significantly higher in women than in men with the disease.

Following is a quote from that study:

"BACKGROUND:

Hashimoto's thyroiditis (HT) is the most common cause of hypothyroidism and is characterized by gradual autoimmune mediated thyroid failure with occasional goiter development. HT is seven times more likely to occur in women than in men.

Papillary thyroid cancer (PTC), the most prevalent form of cancer in the thyroid, is 2.5 times more likely to develop in women than men. Given the relatively high prevalence of these diseases and the increased occurrence in women, we analyzed data from our institution to determine if there is a correlation between Hashimoto's thyroiditis and PTC in women.

METHODS:

From May 1994 to January 2007, 1198 patients underwent thyroid surgery at our institution. Of these, 217 patients were diagnosed with HT (196 women, 21 men). The data from these patients were statistically analyzed using SPSS.

RESULTS:

PTC occurred in 63 of 217 (29%) HT patients and 230 of 981 (23%) patients without HT (P = 0.051). Of these groups, 41 (65%) and 158 (69%) patients, respectively, had tumor sizes >/=1.0 cm; 56/196 women (29%) with HT had coexistent PTC compared with 160/730 women (22%) without HT (P = 0.03). ---

Among women with any type of thyroid malignancy, 56/59 cases (95%) with HT had PTC compared with 159/196 cases (81%) in women without HT (P = 0.006). Additionally, female HT patients with goiters had a significantly lower rate of PTC (9% versus 36%, P < 0.001) compared with women without goiters. These differences were not observed in men with HT.

CONCLUSIONS:

These data demonstrate that HT is associated with an increased risk of developing PTC. Female patients with HT undergoing thyroidectomy are 30% more likely to have PTC. Thus, more aggressive surveillance for PTC may be indicated in patients with HT, especially in women."

Source Link:
http://www.ncbi.nlm.nih.gov/pubmed/17996901
("Hashimoto's thyroiditis a risk factor for papillary thyroid cancer?")

CHAPTER TWO

Can Diet Nutritional Supplementation and Exercise Really Protect Against Thyroid Cancer Risks?

Certainly, a recommendation that is always given to thyroid patients by their doctors is to live the healthiest lives possible, to include proper diet and exercise. The exercise aspect is somewhat obvious and self-explanatory and would include the warning that one should exercise only to tolerance-level and to not overdo when undertaking a regimen, whether of the aerobic or strength and endurance types. Research studies have shown that exercise does indeed lower the risk for cancer development of all types, as does getting proper rest and sleep and so this is one of those obvious things that is available to practically everyone who is healthy enough to exercise regularly.

Research regarding exercise and breast cancer risk reduction (would also obviously apply to other types largely affecting women, including thyroid cancers):

"BACKGROUND:

Epidemiologic evidence strongly suggests that cumulative exposure to ovarian hormones is a determinant of breast cancer risk. Because physical activity can modify menstrual cycle patterns and alter the production of ovarian hormones, it may reduce breast cancer risk; yet few epidemiologic studies have assessed this relationship.

PURPOSE:

The major objective of this study was to determine whether young women (aged 40 and younger) who regularly participated in physical exercise activities during their reproductive years had a reduced risk of breast cancer.

METHODS:

Using a case-control design, we conducted personal interviews of a total of 545 women (aged 40 and younger at diagnosis) who had been newly diagnosed with in situ or invasive breast cancer between July 1, 1983, and January 1, 1989, and a total of 545 control subjects. ---

Cancer: A Great Concern for Thyroid Patients

Case patients and control subjects were individually matched on date of birth (within 36 months), race (white), parity (nulliparous versus parous), and neighborhood of residence. Lifetime histories of participation in physical exercise activities on a regular basis were obtained during the personal interview.

RESULTS:

After adjustment for potential confounding factors, we found that the average number of hours spent in physical exercise activities per week from menarche to 1 year prior to the case patient's diagnosis was a significant predictor of reduced breast cancer risk (two-sided P for trend < .0001). The odds ratio (OR) of breast cancer among women who, on average, spent 3.8 or more hours per week participating in physical exercise activities was 0.42 (95% confidence limits [CLs] = 0.27, 0.64) relative to inactive women. The effect was stronger among women who had had a full-term pregnancy. Comparing most active (> or = 3.8 hours/wk of exercise) women to inactive women, the ORs were 0.28 (95% CL = 0.16, 0.50) for parous and 0.73 (95% CL = 0.38, 1.41) for nulliparous women.---

CONCLUSIONS:

Most previously identified risk factors for breast cancer are reproductive and menstrual events that cannot be readily altered. The protective effect of exercise on breast cancer risk in the women whom we studied suggests that physical activity offers one modifiable lifestyle characteristic that may substantially reduce a woman's lifetime risk of breast cancer.

IMPLICATIONS:

Whether the protective effects of exercise on breast cancer risk are due to alterations in ovarian function and whether they extend into women's menopausal years need to be established. Our results suggest that implementation of regular physical exercise programs as a critical component of a healthy lifestyle should be a high priority for adolescent and adult women."

Source Link:
http://www.ncbi.nlm.nih.gov/pubmed/8072034
("Physical exercise and reduced risk of breast cancer in young women.")

Cancer: A Great Concern for Thyroid Patients

The diet aspect of reducing cancer risk would of course include the recommendation to avoid junk foods (simple carbohydrates -- foods high in saturated fats and high levels of manufactured sugars) and to eat healthy, complex carbohydrates (fruits, vegetables, nuts and grains) however, thyroid patients should avoid certain types of foods that in the long run, can help the thyroid gland to not suffer as severely from autoimmunity that contributes to worsening thyroiditis and hypothyroidism. This would include the avoidance of "goitrogen foods" of which "soy" is a major one and that can be a by-product found in many food-products but is often not recognized unless ingredients are carefully read on food product labels (i.e. soybeans, tofu, soybean oil, soy flour, soy lecithin).

Other goitrogen foods include the following:

- cassava
- Pine nuts
- Peanuts
- Millet
- Strawberries
- Pears
- Peaches ---

- Spinach
- Bamboo shoots
- Sweet Potatoes
- Bok choy
- Broccoli
- Broccolini (Asparations)
- Brussels sprouts
- Cabbage
- Canola
- Cauliflower
- Chinese cabbage
- Choy sum
- Collard greens
- Horseradish
- Kai-lan (Chinese broccoli)
- Kale
- Kohlrabi
- Mizuna
- Mustard greens
- Radishes
- Rapeseed (yu choy)
- Rapini
- Rutabagas
- Tatsoi
- Turnips

Some medical sources state that the goitrogen effect of these foods, can be reduced considerably when they are cooked properly (those that require cooking) and when those who have thyroid disease, consume them in moderation (especially those foods that don't require being cooked).

Healthy versus Unhealthy Fats

An additional note in regard to "saturated fats" as mentioned previously -- these are the unhealthy dietary types, while there are healthy dietary fats called "monounsaturated and polyunsaturated" and these actually help to lower any bad fat levels in the body that can lead to high cholesterol.

One method for making sure that one is taking ample amounts of healthy fat in the diet is by supplementing with "omega-3 fats" (fish oil) found in over-the-counter caplets available in the natural supplements departments of department stores and health shops. This can help to raise the "HDL" cholesterol level (the healthy type), which can decrease any harmful effects from elevated "LDL" cholesterol levels (the unhealthy type).

Following is a research study quote, in regard to healthy cholesterol levels, decreasing prostrate cancer risks in males and how statin medications may help in this area, when needed (logically also true of other cancers including thyroid types):

"BACKGROUND:

Studies suggest a decreased risk of high-grade prostate cancer in men with lower circulating total cholesterol and that statins may protect against aggressive disease. Confirmation in additional populations and examination of associations for lipoprotein subfractions are needed.

METHODS:

We examined prostate cancer risk and serum total and HDL cholesterol in the ATBC Study cohort (n = 29,093). Cox proportional hazards models were used to estimate the relative risk of total (n = 2,041), non-aggressive (n = 829), aggressive (n = 461), advanced (n = 412), and high-grade (n = 231) prostate cancer by categories of total and HDL cholesterol.

Cancer: A Great Concern for Thyroid Patients

RESULTS:

After excluding the first 10 years of follow-up, men with higher serum total cholesterol were at increased risk of overall ($\geq$240 vs. <200 mg/dl: HR = 1.22, 95% CI 1.03-1.44, p-trend = 0.01) and advanced ($\geq$240 vs. <200 mg/dl: HR = 1.85, 95% CI 1.13-3.03, p-trend = 0.05) prostate cancer. Higher HDL cholesterol was suggestively associated with a decreased risk of prostate cancer regardless of stage or grade.

CONCLUSIONS:

In this population of smokers, high serum total cholesterol was associated with higher risk of advanced prostate cancer, and high HDL cholesterol suggestively reduced the risk of prostate cancer overall. These results support previous studies and, indirectly, support the hypothesis that statins may reduce the risk of advanced prostate cancer by lowering cholesterol."
Source Link:
http://www.ncbi.nlm.nih.gov/pubmed/21915616
("Serum total and HDL cholesterol and risk of prostate cancer.")

Cancer: A Great Concern for Thyroid Patients

Other Healthy Supplements that Decrease Thyroid Cancer Risk

According to a great deal of medical research that is available, nutritional supplements can indeed offset the risk for cancer development of all types. Some studies have shown that essential vitamins becoming deficient can significantly increase the chances for cancer developing.

This includes a vitamin that has become deficient in the American public as well as in third world countries of the world and this would be the all-important "vitamin D" (also considered an essential steroid).

Here is one research study from Pubmed/U.S. NIH, to this effect:

*"**PURPOSE:***

Higher serum levels of the main circulating form of vitamin D, 25-hydroxyvitamin D (25(OH)D), are associated with substantially lower incidence rates of colon, breast, ovarian, renal, pancreatic, aggressive prostate and other cancers.

METHODS:

Epidemiological findings combined with newly discovered mechanisms suggest a new model of cancer etiology that accounts for these actions of 25(OH)D and calcium. Its seven phases are disjunction, initiation, natural selection, overgrowth, metastasis, involution, and transition (abbreviated DINOMIT). Vitamin D metabolites prevent disjunction of cells and are beneficial in other phases.

RESULTS/CONCLUSIONS:

It is projected that raising the minimum year-around serum 25(OH)D level to 40 to 60 ng/mL (100-150 nmol/L) would prevent approximately 58,000 new cases of breast cancer and 49,000 new cases of colorectal cancer each year, and three fourths of deaths from these diseases in the United States and Canada, based on observational studies combined with a randomized trial. Such intakes also are expected to reduce case-fatality rates of patients who have breast, colorectal, or prostate cancer by half. ---

There are no unreasonable risks from intake of 2000 IU per day of vitamin D(3), or from a population serum 25(OH)D level of 40 to 60 ng/mL. The time has arrived for nationally coordinated action to substantially increase intake of vitamin D and calcium. "

Source Link:
http://www.ncbi.nlm.nih.gov/pubmed/19523595 ("Vitamin D for cancer prevention: global perspective.")

Note that this research states that taking up to "2,000 IU of vitamin D per day", is not considered over-supplementation however, many doctors recommend approximately "1,000 IU per day", unless a severe deficiency is found and in these cases, mega-doses may be required for a period of time.

Getting Blood Tested for Nutritional Deficiencies

All thyroid patients should undergo testing of major vitamin levels (i.e. D, B12, E and B6) and other nutrients.

This includes minerals, protein and electrolyte levels, because deficiencies can be present without necessarily causing any suggestive symptoms. If vitamin levels or other nutrients are found to be deficient, further testing should also be done, to find if there are malabsorption syndromes present as well. These are disorders, in which nutrients are hindered in the body and organs cannot utilize them properly, which can include the digestive tract and the liver.

Diseases of these organs, resulting in nutritional malabsorption, can include Celiac disease (intolerance to gluten in the diet) and types of liver disease, such as viral and autoimmune hepatitis. If such diseases are found, supplementation with the needed nutrients that are deficient, in addition to treating the underlying disease process would become necessary. If deficiencies-only are found, with no particular cause behind them (idiopathic), supplementing them to bring them back up to proper levels, can be highly beneficial, not only as a cancer preventative but for overall better health as well.

CHAPTER THREE

Supplementing with Selenium

One nutrient that has also been covered in medical research studies, regarding supplements that can decrease thyroid disease activity, is "selenium", which is both a mineral and an electrolyte that is essential in the body. According to these research studies, the mineral actually "modifies" levels of the antibodies that cause thyroid diseases as discussed earlier. The two major thyroid antibodies, also called "auto-antibodies", that attack key proteins within the gland, causing diseases such as Hashimoto's thyroiditis and Graves' disease, are the "anti-thyroidperoxidase" (immune cells that attack the thyroidperoxidase enzyme/protein – abbreviated "Anti-TPO") and the "anti-thyroglobulin" (immune cells that attack the thyroglobulin enzyme/protein – abbreviated anti-TG).

Selenium, supplemented as a daily regimen, is cited in these studies as having the ability to reduce the TPO antibodies, thereby reducing disease activity in the thyroid gland and the associated inflammation that is also involved.

Cancer: A Great Concern for Thyroid Patients

Additionally, other research studies state that it can also reduce the risk for cancers of the lung, colorectal, and prostate types.

Research citing selenium as a cancer risk reducer:

"Studies examining the relationship between dietary selenium intake and risk of various cancers have shown that low selenium intake is associated with higher cancer rates. A recent well-controlled intervention trial studied whether selenium supplementation can prevent cancer in subjects who have a history of skin cancer and live in areas of the United States with low soil selenium levels. Selenium supplementation did not reduce skin cancer rates, but the incidence of total, lung, colorectal, and prostate cancers was significantly reduced by the intervention. Although these data need confirmation, they suggest that adequate selenium intake is essential for cancer prevention."

Source Link:
http://www.ncbi.nlm.nih.gov/pubmed/9279064
("Dietary selenium repletion may reduce cancer incidence in people at high risk who live in areas with low soil selenium.")

Research citing selenium as a modifier of thyroid autoimmunity activity:

"In areas with severe selenium deficiency there is a higher incidence of thyroiditis due to a decreased activity of selenium-dependent glutathione peroxidase activity within thyroid cells. Selenium-dependent enzymes also have several modifying effects on the immune system. Therefore, even mild selenium deficiency may contribute to the development and maintenance of autoimmune thyroid diseases.

We performed a blinded, placebo-controlled, prospective study in female patients (n = 70; mean age, 47.5 +/- 0.7 yr) with autoimmune thyroiditis and thyroid peroxidase antibodies (TPOAb) and/or Tg antibodies (TgAb) above 350 IU/ml. The primary end point of the study was the change in TPOAb concentrations. Secondary end points were changes in TgAb, TSH, and free thyroid hormone levels as well as ultrasound pattern of the thyroid and quality of life estimation.

Patients were randomized into 2 age- and antibody (TPOAb)-matched groups; 36 patients received 200 microg (2.53 micromol) sodium selenite/d, orally, for 3 months, and 34 patients received placebo. All patients were substituted with L-T(4) to maintain TSH within the normal range. TPOAb, TgAb, TSH, and free thyroid hormones were determined by commercial assays. The echogenicity of the thyroid was monitored with high resolution ultrasound. The mean TPOAb concentration decreased significantly to 63.6% (P = 0.013) in the selenium group vs. 88% (P = 0.95) in the placebo group.

A subgroup analysis of those patients with TPOAb greater than 1200 IU/ml revealed a mean 40% reduction in the selenium-treated patients compared with a 10% increase in TPOAb in the placebo group. TgAb concentrations were lower in the placebo group at the beginning of the study and significantly further decreased (P = 0.018), but were unchanged in the selenium group.

Nine patients in the selenium-treated group had completely normalized antibody concentrations, in contrast to two patients in the placebo group (by chi(2) test, P = 0.01). ---

Cancer: A Great Concern for Thyroid Patients

Ultrasound of the thyroid showed normalized echogenicity in these patients. The mean TSH, free T(4), and free T(3) levels were unchanged in both groups. We conclude that selenium substitution may improve the inflammatory activity in patients with autoimmune thyroiditis, especially in those with high activity.

Whether this effect is specific for autoimmune thyroiditis or may also be effective in other endocrine autoimmune diseases has yet to be investigated."

Source Link: http://www.ncbi.nlm.nih.gov/pubmed/11932302 (Selenium supplementation in patients with autoimmune thyroiditis decreases thyroid peroxidase antibodies concentrations.")

The conclusions that can be derived from the combination of these two previously quoted medical studies, is that both thyroid autoimmunity and cancers that can potentially affect the thyroid gland, can both be modified and/or reduced in risk for development, through selenium supplementation.

It is always recommended however, that dosing directions are followed according to a manufacturer's label and that the supplement is reported to one's doctor, to make sure it cannot potentially contraindicate (interfere or interact significantly) with other medications or supplements that are already being taken.

CHAPTER FOUR

Monitoring for Thyroid Cancer Symptoms

The symptoms of thyroid cancer can be non-specific and often, there are no symptoms to indicate that the disease is present. When symptoms do occur, they usually involve discomfort of various types, in the throat. A person with thyroid malignancy developing may find that they are having throat pain that can be felt when turning their head or stretching their neck with body position changes and/or they may feel soreness inside their throat that manifests like a typical sore throat that occurs with colds, viral illnesses or allergies. The difference being that a sore throat that occurs with thyroid cancer does not usually get better but will worsen over time. Thyroid cancer can also cause voice changes such as hoarseness or a deeper tone to one's voice due to any constriction present from swelling or tumors requiring more effort to project words. When thyroid tumors, also called "nodules" increase in size with malignancy, they can cause a person to experience difficulty swallowing or even breathing difficulties if they become large enough.

Cancer: A Great Concern for Thyroid Patients

Other than these aforementioned symptoms affecting the throat, other indirect symptoms of thyroid malignancy can occur rarely, including fever or anemia (if blood loss is involved) but in many cases, the disease develops with no noticeable symptoms being present.

Self Palpating (Examining) the Thyroid Gland

With the fact of thyroid cancer not causing symptoms in many cases, thyroid disease patients can perform home self-exams, of their glands and report any noticeable changes in size or texture that may occur within it, to their doctors. While a person can sometimes detect a goiter and/or thyroid nodules by self examination, a definitive diagnoses must be given by a qualified physician.

Abnormalities in size and/or texture of the thyroid gland can occur with both hypothyroid and hyperthyroid conditions but are more common in autoimmune thyroid diseases. As previously stated, this can also be the case with thyroid malignancy as well. If a person is experiencing thyroid-related symptoms or they have detected an abnormal feeling in their thyroid gland, a preliminary self-examination can be done.

An appointment with a qualified physician should also be scheduled.

A patient can then report any findings that indicate problems in the gland to his medical doctor. The eMedicine/WebMD website states in their article titled "Goiter Nontoxic: Follow-Up", under the Patient Education sub-heading that "Thyroid self-examination may be taught to patients, allowing them to monitor their own body for early changes in gland size."

Palpating the Thyroid Gland

A person can feel his own throat, using the fingertips (palpation), in the area of the thyroid gland, to detect swelling or lumps. The thyroid is located in the center of the throat, directly beneath the Adams apple, which in males is more prominent but can usually be located easily in females as well. Once finding the Adams apple, the isthmus (middle portion) of the thyroid is only about an inch or, slightly lower below it and will be slightly raised. If the isthmus protrudes significantly, or feels very firm to the touch, this can indicate a goiter or thyroid nodule being present in that portion of the gland.

Cancer: A Great Concern for Thyroid Patients

Shape of the Gland

There are also two lobes of the thyroid gland, one on each side of it, that extend about an inch toward the inside of the throat and that extend upward toward the Adams apple, about even with it. The gland is typically small and forms a butterfly shape. The lobes actually attach to the Adams apple and throat with connecting cartilage and tissue but when they are normal size, are usually not easily felt unless pressed-on firmly with the fingertips. If they are easily detectable without firmly pressing down on them or are visible without the need to palpate them, this can indicate a goiter or nodules in the lobe-areas as well.

The Swallow Test

While palpation is being done to detect swelling (enlargement) in the gland, any lumps or protrusions that might indicate a thyroid nodule (tumor-like growth) or several of them should also be checked for. These can also be spotted by tilting the head back, while looking in a mirror and taking sips of water.

With this method, one can watch for any signs of enlargement or lumps as the gland moves up and down in the throat. Some people with enlarged glands are found to have both goiter and nodules, which is referred to as a "nodular goiter" or a "multi-nodular goiter".

Difficulty Swallowing

If a person feels a lump on the inside of their throat when swallowing, this can indicate a thyroid nodule that is growing toward the inside and that cannot be felt from the outside of the throat. If there is a general feeling of difficulty swallowing or breathing due to the throat being constricted, this may also indicate a goiter in which the enlargement is swelling toward the inside of the throat. This type problem is not always indicative of thyroid problems but can be related to esophagus problems as well.

If any of these self-examination methods are found to indicate a problem in the gland, it should be reported to a medical doctor as soon as possible for further evaluation.

Thyroid Cancer Diagnostic Tests

While blood abnormalities would actually be considered a "sign" rather than a "symptom" of thyroid cancer, there are several of these that can be ordered for someone suspected of having possibly malignancy in their thyroid gland. These tests would include a "Complete Blood Count", which evaluates the red and white blood cells, to see if there is a decrease or change in the size of them.

With cancer of any kind the total white blood cell count (leukocytes) will often increase, which is a condition known as "leukocytosis" or with certain types of cancer, it may actually decrease (i.e. with lymphoma and leukemia), which is referred to as "leukopenia". Adversely the total red blood cells (erythrocytes) may decrease if blood loss has begun to occur with cancers of any kind (anemia). Inflammatory markers in the blood can increase when cancer is present as well but may also do-so simply due to highly active thyroid autoimmunity (i.e. C-Reactive Protein and the Erythrocyte Sedimentation Rate levels).

Two blood tests that are more specific to thyroid cancer diagnosis are the "calcitonin" and "thyroglobulin" levels. These substances will become elevated in the blood, in some cases of thyroid cancer types. They are also used for follow-up tests after treatment for thyroid malignancy has been administered to monitor progress of the treatment.

In some cases, a thyroid biopsy will be performed to detect or to rule out cancer being present within the gland. Some patients are given a "fine needle aspiration" biopsy, which is usually an out-patient test in which a hypodermic needle is inserted into the gland, to extract small amounts of tissue for analysis. Other patients may be referred for a surgical biopsy in which a larger area of tissue is removed while they are under full anesthesia. Yet other patients may be sent for imaging tests of their thyroid glands, such as "thyroid ultrasound" and "MRI" (magnetic resonance imaging) or a "CT Scan" (multiple-angle radiograph images).

CHAPTER FIVE

Thyroid Cancer Treatments

When a patient is confirmed as having thyroid cancer, via the medical tests that diagnose it, the treating doctor will refer the patient to a surgeon, who will determine how the cancer will need to be removed. If the cancer affects only one of the two lobes of the thyroid, the surgeon may wish to perform what is called a "lobectomy", (partial thyroidectomy) meaning there will be removal of only one side of the gland.

If the surgeon feels removal of only one lobe, still places the patient at risk for the cancer returning, he may instead decide to remove the entire gland, which is referred to as a "total thyroidectomy".

The type surgery is also determined by considering the type of thyroid cancer that is involved. Some types of cancer are more aggressive than others and with these the surgeon will always recommend total thyroid removal. Surgeons also must determine at what stage the cancer is in, meaning how far it has progressed.

In order to decrease the risk of the cancer returning, the surgeon may also want to remove the lymph nodes in the neck, that are located near the thyroid gland. The lymph nodes may also be sent off for laboratory analysis to determine if they already contained cancer, which might then lead the surgeon to recommend further treatment(s).

Post Operative Thyroid Cancer Treatments

Additional treatment after any type of thyroidectomy might also include Radio Active Iodine Therapy (RAI) or Chemotherapy, to destroy any remaining thyroid tissue that is capable of absorbing iodine in the body or any remaining cancer cells.

Any remaining thyroid tissue that is capable of taking up iodine, which is what the thyroid mainly consists of, also has the ability to re-develop cancer cells and is the reason RAI is sometimes used following a Total Thyroidectomy. Chemotherapy is directed at any remaining cancer cells that might remain in the body after a Total Thyroidectomy.

Regardless of the type of thyroid surgery that is performed, thyroid hormone replacement therapy is always used following thyroid cancer surgeries. The goal of the hormone therapy is to suppress the patient's increased TSH level, which decreases when thyroid hormone is elevated back to normal levels via a prescribed hormone replacement dose (hypothyroid therapy). This also helps prevent recurrence of cancer but also replaces any hormone the thyroid gland is not capable of producing following surgery (hypothyroidism).

If a patient is given RAI after surgery, they may not be replaced with thyroid hormone for a month or two following the treatment. Most patients will need thyroid hormone replacement therapy following any type of thyroidectomy, as lifelong treatment.

The treating Doctor will prescribe a starting dose of thyroid hormone for the patient and will order follow-up blood re-testing to adjust the dose to the correct level over time, which is called "titrating" the dose. Each new dose level takes about eight weeks to fully adjust in the body.

Following are helpful suggestions for patients who are placed on thyroid hormone therapy following thyroid cancer treatment:

• Take your thyroid hormone medication on an empty stomach, with plenty of water.
• Take your thyroid hormone medication at the same time each day.
• If you take vitamins or supplements containing iron or calcium, be sure to take them six hours apart from your thyroid medication dose.
• When you have blood retests of your thyroid hormone levels, take your medication at the same time, to correlate with each blood draw.
• Never adjust your own thyroid medication dose.

Thyroid cancers have a very high treatment success rate but that success rate is even higher when thyroid cancers are diagnosed and treated as early as possible.
It is very important to see your doctor if you discover any nodules (tumor-like growths) on your thyroid gland or if you have difficulty swallowing, a chronic sore throat or feel, that you might have a growth on the inside of your throat.

(END)

About the Author:

I am a husband, father, grandfather and lifetime contract salesman, with experience in health writing that began in 2004. I completed theological studies with Liberty University in 1996. I formerly served as editor and forum moderator of Thyroid Health for a major multi-topic content site and as a general health writer for another, where I received Editor's Choice Awards for my articles on health subjects.

In 2003 I was diagnosed with hypothyroidism; "Hashimoto's thyroiditis" being the cause. This autoimmune form of thyroid disease that causes destruction of the thyroid gland resulted in my also developing "Chronic Fatigue Syndrome", due to a compromised immune system with severe co-morbid "Adrenal Fatigue".

I also suffered severe anxiety symptoms, including panic attacks early into the onset of Hashimoto's thyroiditis (Hashitoxicosis). A common, benign heart murmur I was diagnosed with in my teens called "Mitral Valve Prolapse", also worsened in severity of symptoms, with the development of these other health disorders.

Cancer: A Great Concern for Thyroid Patients

My eventual receiving of diagnoses was a difficult process with proper diagnostic testing not being ordered by the first doctors I sought treatment from. These types of issues were inspiration for me to become proactive in my own health care and to self-educate myself on these health disorders, which I have done extensively since 2003.

I now enjoy sharing this information with other patients experiencing my same health disorders.

www.ingramcontent.com/pod-product-compliance
Lightning Source LLC
Chambersburg PA
CBHW061230280526
45784CB00006B/2711